Treat Your Own Carpal Tunnel Syndrome

Treatment and Prevention Strategies for
Individuals, Therapists, and Employers

by
Jim Johnson, PT

Drawings by Eunice Johnson

Why Is The Print In This Book So Big?

People who read my books sometimes wonder why the print is so big in many of them. Some tend to think it's because I'm trying to make a little book bigger or a short book longer.

Actually, the main reason I use bigger print is for the same reason I intentionally write short books, usually under 100 pages–it's just plain easier to read and get the information quicker!

You see, the books I write address common, everyday problems that people of *all* ages have. In other words, the "typical" reader of my books could be a teenager, a busy housewife, a CEO, a construction worker, or a retired senior citizen with poor eyesight. Therefore, by writing books with larger print that are short and to the point, *everyone* can get the information quickly and with ease. After all, what good is a book full of useful information if nobody ever finishes it?

I have given my best effort to ensure that this book is entirely based upon scientific evidence and not on intuition, single case reports, opinions of authorities, anecdotal evidence, or unsystematic clinical observations. Where I do state my opinion in this book, it is directly stated as such.

—*Jim Johnson, P.T.*

Table of Contents

What Exactly Is
The Carpal Tunnel?

The best way to solve a problem is to first *understand* it. Then, once you know exactly what's going on, you can find an effective way to *get rid of it*. Since I don't know what you already know about carpal tunnel syndrome, I'm going to start at the *very* beginning.

The Median Nerve

In carpal tunnel syndrome, you have a problem with a nerve in your wrist. The nerve is called the *median* nerve. It's actually a pretty long nerve though, and goes all the way down your whole arm. Let's have a look…

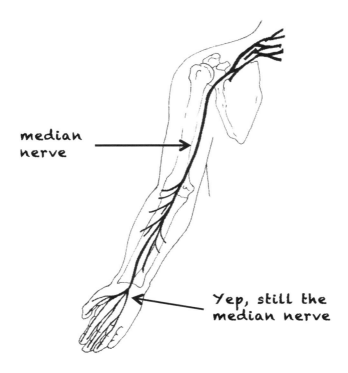

median
nerve

Yep, still the
median nerve

Figure 1. The median nerve. Note how it runs down your whole arm.

You can see from the picture that the median nerve isn't just a nerve in the wrist, it's actually like a long string of spaghetti that starts out at your shoulder - and ends up all the way down in the hand. A close-up shows us that this median nerve is really a pretty complicated structure…

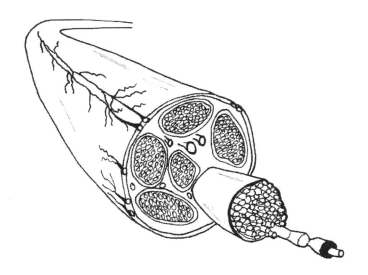

Figure 2. Close-up of the median nerve.

Note how the median nerve is made up of many different "bundles" of fibers. Some of these you see are *sensory* fibers – meaning that they carry sensations you feel such as pain or tingling. Yet other fibers are *motor* fibers – meaning they carry signals that tell your muscles to move. This is why the median nerve is called a *mixed nerve* – because it is made up of both sensory *and* motor fibers. In practical terms, this means that if something were to put pressure on the median nerve in your wrist area, you could feel funny sensations (because of pressure on the *sensory* fibers) and/or you could have a weak finger (because of pressure on the *motor* fibers).

The Carpal Tunnel

The next thing to know about the median nerve is that it goes through *the carpal tunnel.*

So what exactly is it? Taking the name apart, you know what a tunnel is, but what's the heck is a carpal? Well, it's not as fancy as the name sounds – carpals are just the medical word for your *wrist bones.* You've got a bunch of them, here's what they look like...

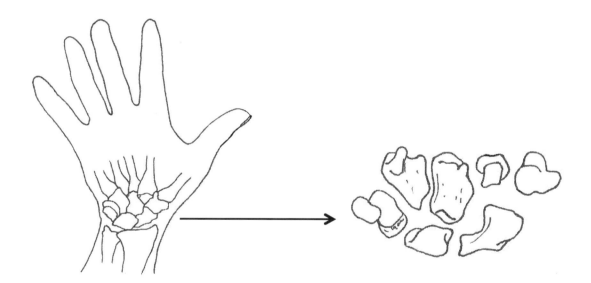

Figure 3. The right hand, palm up. Where the wrist bones (carpals) sit.

Figure 4. What the tiny carpals look like separated from each other.

Now the carpal bones you see above make up only *half* of the carpal tunnel – think of them as being the "floor" of the carpal tunnel. The "roof", on the other hand, isn't made of bone, but of a softer structure called the *transverse carpal ligament.* On the next page is a picture of it...

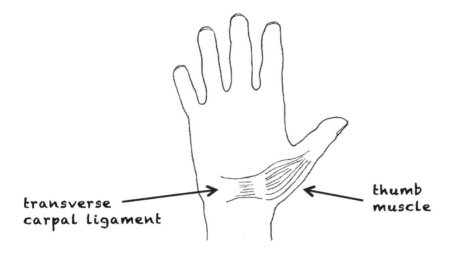

Figure 5. The right hand, palm up - the transverse carpal ligament.

As you can see, the transverse carpal ligament (also called the flexor retinaculum – try saying that tens times) isn't a particularly exciting looking structure. It's really like a big piece of tape stretched across your wrist that helps support it and hold things together. Of note, when surgeons do a carpal tunnel release, this is the ligament they cut apart.

Anyway, when you put these two structures together, the carpal bones as the "floor", and the transverse carpal ligament as the "roof", you have what has popularly become known as "the carpal tunnel"...

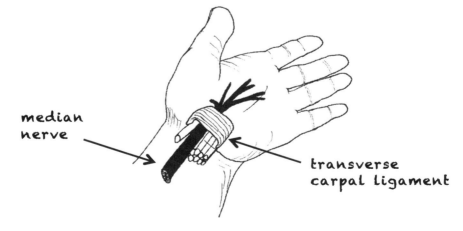

Figure 6. Overhead view of the carpal tunnel -- formed by the transverse carpal ligament (the roof) and the carpal bones (the floor) hidden underneath.

You'll notice there's some stuff packed in the carpal tunnel. The median nerve you can see, but what are all those other little things? Well, let's look at a cross-sectional view - as if we're looking right *into* the carpal tunnel...

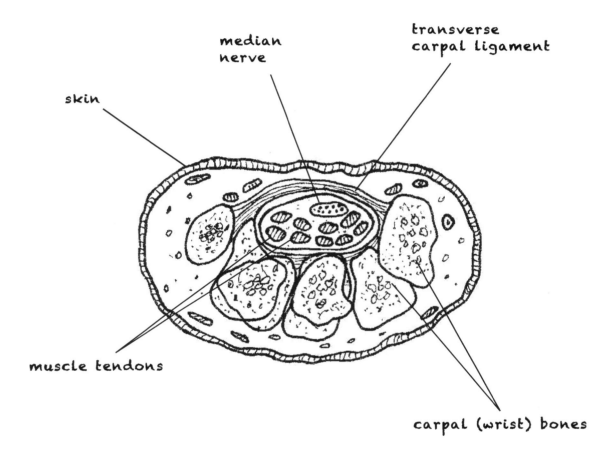

Figure 7. Cross-sectional view of the carpal tunnel and the stuff inside.

As you can see, the carpal tunnel contains the median nerve and nine *tendons.* What do tendons do? Tendons connect muscles to bones, and these particular nine tendons attach directly to muscles that move your fingers. Notice how they are *right next* to the median nerve.

So that's the carpal tunnel and the major parts inside it. Up next you're going to learn exactly what is going on in the carpal tunnel that's got that median nerve all worked up.

Quick Review

- ✓ carpal tunnel syndrome involves a problem with the median nerve

- ✓ the median nerve isn't just in the wrist – rather it's a long nerve that runs *all* the way down your arm

- ✓ while it looks like a piece of spaghetti, the median nerve is a mixed nerve - it contains both *sensory* and *motor* fibers.

- ✓ the carpal tunnel is made up of a roof (the transverse carpal ligament), and a floor (the carpal bones)

- ✓ the main structures in the carpal tunnel are the median nerve and nine finger tendons

---

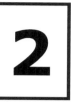 What Causes Carpal Tunnel Syndrome?

People who have carpal tunnel syndrome most commonly complain of an unpleasant tingling, burning or numbness sensation in certain areas of their hand and fingers...

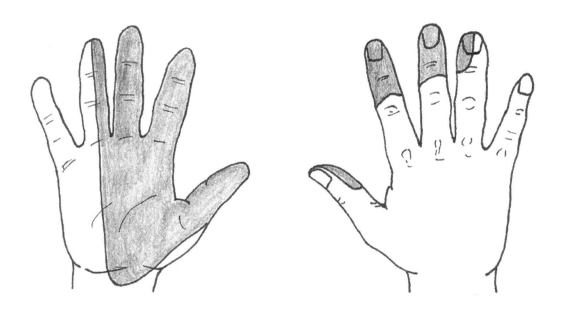

Figure 8. Shaded areas show the most common places where people feel carpal tunnel symptoms of burning, tingling and numbness.

If you look at the fingers, these symptoms are in some pretty specific spots – the thumb, index finger, middle finger, *and only the side of the ring finger.* Why?

A quick look at where the median travels in the hand tells the whole story...

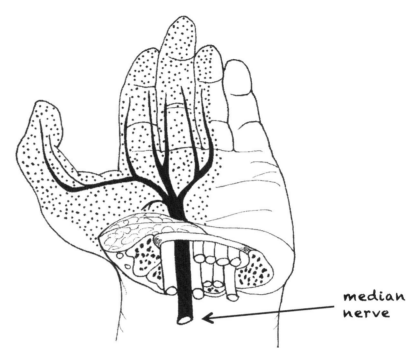

Figure 9. The left hand – palm up. Where the median nerve goes into the hand and fingers. Dots show areas where symptoms are felt.

Because the median nerve only goes to *certain* fingers, those are usually the ones where the tingling, burning, and numbness are felt. Which brings up the million-dollar question – what makes the median nerve cause these symptoms?

The Not Too Common Causes of Carpal Tunnel Syndrome

If I was to give someone the short answer as to what causes carpal tunnel syndrome, I would say, "Increased pressure on the median nerve."

You'll notice I said *increased* pressure. Just as there is a normal amount of pressure in your arteries, this you know as your "blood pressure", there is also is a normal amount of pressure being exerted on the median nerve *every* day as it sits in the carpal tunnel – that it lives just fine with.

The trouble begins when the pressure increases repeatedly or stays elevated – and there are many things that can cause this. To name a few…

- a wrist *fracture* can increase carpal tunnel pressure

- swelling from fluid retention during *pregnancy* can increase carpal tunnel pressure

- a condition known as *amyloidosis* can produce amyloid deposits in the carpal tunnel and increase pressure

So there *are* some cases where doctors can figure out the exact reason for the increased carpal tunnel pressure. Unfortunately, *most* cases of carpal tunnel syndrome aren't that clear-cut…

Idiopathic Carpal Tunnel Syndrome?

When you have carpal tunnel syndrome, and there is no obvious reason, doctors say you have *idiopathic* carpal tunnel syndrome. This means that while they know you have carpal tunnel syndrome, they can't say positively, absolutely, 100% for sure what caused it.

However, if you dig around in the research like I have, you will find an awful lot of clues about the likely sequence of events that causes carpal tunnel syndrome in the majority of people…

Smaller Than Normal Carpal Tunnels

Did you know that many people with carpal tunnel syndrome have *much smaller* carpal tunnels than normal? And this means that they have much less room to spare *if* something in the carpal tunnel does get irritated or swollen. Here are a few studies that have shown this...

- one study took MRI scans of 20 wrists with carpal tunnel syndrome and compared them to 20 wrists of healthy volunteers (Horch 1997). Results showed that the cross-sectional area of the carpal tunnel was much smaller in those who suffered with carpal tunnel syndrome.

- 14 male patients with idiopathic carpal tunnel syndrome were compared to 26 normal male controls (Papaioannou 1992). CT scans were taken of their carpal tunnels. The proximal part of the carpal tunnel in patients was found to be smaller than the pain-free controls.

- In this study, 11 female patients with idiopathic carpal tunnel syndrome were compared to 26 normal male and female controls (Gelmers 1981). X-rays showed that the patients had much narrower carpal tunnels compared to the controls.

- The cross-sectional area of the carpal tunnel was measured in 26 women with idiopathic carpal tunnel syndrome by CT scans and compared to 19 normal females (Dekel 1980). Once again, the women with carpal tunnel syndrome had much smaller carpal tunnels than the control group that was pain-free.

As you can see, whether researchers use an MRI, CT-scan, or X-ray, it's a quite consistent finding in the literature that people who suffer from *idiopathic* carpal tunnel syndrome – males and females alike – all have a tendency to have much smaller sized carpal tunnel than those who don't suffer from it. So the cards might have not been stacked in a person's favor to begin with.

Repeated Wrist Movements

Yet another big factor in getting idiopathic carpal tunnel syndrome is the way people use their hands and wrists. Many individuals who get carpal tunnel syndrome put their wrists through repeated *flexion* and *extension* motions. What's wrist flexion and extension? Take a look...

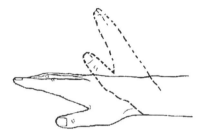

Figure 10. Extension is when you bring your wrist *up*.

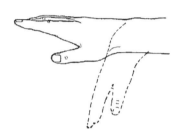

Figure 11. Flexion is when you bend your wrist *down*.

So what's bending your wrist up and down got to do with getting carpal tunnel syndrome?

It's like this: *these two motions actually change the shape of your carpal tunnel as the wrist moves* – that is, the cross sectional area of the carpal tunnel actually gets *smaller* with flexion and extension of the wrist. It's a fact...

- a 1997 study used MRI to examine 20 wrists that had carpal tunnel syndrome and 20 wrists of healthy volunteers (Horch 1997). Researchers noted that in all subjects, the carpal tunnel got much *smaller* when subjects flexed or extended their wrists. Other studies have found the same results (Yoshioka 1993).

Problem is, making your carpal tunnel smaller *drives up the pressure in the carpal tunnel.* Thus, you're actually making the pressure go *up* in your wrist as you're bending it up or down. This too has been proven to occur...

- one study measured carpal tunnel pressure in 103 patients with idiopathic carpal tunnel syndrome, as well as 25 normal control subjects (Sanz 2005). Measurements were taken with the wrist in extension, flexion, and straight positions. In both patients and control subjects, carpal tunnel pressure rose when the wrist was placed in flexion and extension. The lowest recorded pressures occurred with the wrist was held straight. Other researchers have found the same thing (Luchetti 2008).

I also need to mention that there are a few other things you might be doing with your hands that drive up carpal tunnel pressure as well...

- in an interesting study, researchers recorded the pressure in the carpal tunnel during nine different functional positions of the hand and wrist in 72 people with carpal tunnel syndrome, and 21 control subjects (Seradge 1995). In both controls *and* patients, a significant rise in pressure was noted when making a fist, holding objects, and pressing the fingers against resistance (like typing).

It Gets Worse

As if it's not enough that the pressure goes up in the carpal tunnel when you flex and extend your wrist, something else happens too – *the circulation decreases to your hand...*

- researchers measured the blood flow to the hand in 22 patients with carpal tunnel and 12 healthy volunteers as they flexed and extended their wrists (Ozcan 2011). Doppler studies of the radial and ulnar arteries (the major blood suppliers of the hand) showed that blood flow *decreased* to the hand when *both* patients and volunteers extended and flexed their wrists.

So we see the effects that repeated wrist motions have on the carpal tunnel – the pressure goes up and the circulation goes down. Although these changes occur only temporarily as you flex or extend your wrist, doing them *repeatedly* could set forth *two* likely chain of events...

Chain of Events #1

Increased pressure in the carpal tunnel from repeated wrist motions in turn puts increased pressure on the median nerve itself. Looking back at the picture of the median nerve, notice that there are blood vessels on its outside...

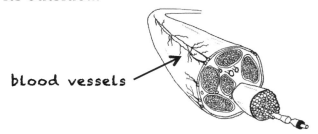

Figure 12. The median nerve

These blood vessels carry much needed nutrients and such to the nerve – and when the pressure goes up in the carpal tunnel, the flow of blood through these tiny vessels is not as good as it should be. Among other things, this can cause the median nerve to swell, which is exactly what we find in people with carpal tunnel syndrome...

- the size of the median nerve (cross-sectional area) was measured by ultrasound in 30 patients with carpal tunnel syndrome and 30 healthy volunteers (Guan 2011). Researchers found that the median nerve in the carpal tunnel syndrome patients was much bigger compared to normal subjects. Other researchers have also found swelling of the median nerve in carpal tunnel patients compared to controls using ultrasound (Sernik 2008) and MRI's (Uchiyama 2005 and Cudlip 2002).

And a swollen nerve is an aggravated nerve that could then start to give you the symptoms of carpal tunnel syndrome.

Chain of Events #2

The second chain of events that can cause carpal tunnel symptoms also has to do with the flow of blood - and builds on everything we've been talking about. Here's a diagram to make is easy to follow...

a person bends their wrist

↓

carpal tunnel pressure goes up

↓

blood flow decreases to the carpal tunnel

↓

person straightens their wrist

↓

carpal tunnel pressure goes back down

↓

blood flow returns to normal

↓

therefore, bending and then straightening the wrist over and over again causes the flow of blood to increase, and then decrease in the carpal tunnel

↓

this can cause what is known as an *ischemic-reperfusion injury*

At this point, you're probably thinking, "What's an ischemic-reperfusion injury?" Well, unfortunately, it's not something you hear about too often when people talk about carpal tunnel syndrome – but it should be.

Simply put, an ischemic-reperfusion injury is the damage caused when blood returns to an area after a period of *ischemia* or restricted blood flow. For instance, if I tie a rope tightly around your leg, your foot isn't going to get a lot of blood going to it (ischemia). However when I untie the rope, blood flows back into your foot (reperfusion), and your foot feels much better.

Of course most of the time, the return of blood flow is a good thing, but sometimes all that blood rushing back in actually *injures* the tissues – and then we have an *ischemic-reperfusion injury*. And why exactly does the return of blood cause injury when it should be welcomed? Well, it's kind of complicated, and too detailed to go into here, but let's just say it has to do with inflammation and oxidative stress.

The bigger question, however, is how do we *really* know that there's an ischemic-reperfusion injury going on in the carpal tunnel that's causing problems?

Well, evidence that this type of injury is actually occurring comes from studies where researchers take tissue samples from the wrists of people with carpal tunnel - and find high levels of substances that are associated with this type of injury, substances such as cytokines and MDA (malondialdehyde).

In other words, if this type of injury *is* actually taking place in the carpal tunnel, then we should be able to find traces that it is happening - which we have...

- tissue samples were taken from the tendons in the carpal tunnel of 41 patients with idiopathic carpal tunnel syndrome, and compared to controls that had no history of carpal tunnel (Freeland 2002). Results showed that carpal tunnel patients had a *two-fold* increase of malondialdehyde, and *three* times the level of the cytokine IL-6 than the control tissue samples. Other researchers who have done similar studies have also found increased levels of malondialdehyde and the cytokine IL-6 compared to controls (Tucci 1997).

So we have good evidence in the medical literature that an ischemic-reperfusion injury *is* actually taking place in the wrists of people with carpal tunnel syndrome. But as this occurs, what kind of damage does it cause that could create carpal tunnel symptoms, such as pain and tingling in the hands?

Well, over time, an ischemic-reperfusion injury can cause *two* major changes to take place. The first one is that the median nerve becomes *fibrotic* over time, that is the body is forming *extra* connective tissue *on* the nerve...

- a 2005 study examined 31 hands with carpal tunnel as they underwent surgery (Tuncali 2005). Surgeons noted that the more severe the carpal tunnel syndrome, the more fibrosis was found.

The second major change that can be caused by an ischemic-reperfusion injury, takes place in the *subsynovial connective tissue*. And what's the subsynovial connective tissue? It's basically just a type of tissue that sits just above the tendons in the carpal tunnel. Here's a drawing to give you a better idea...

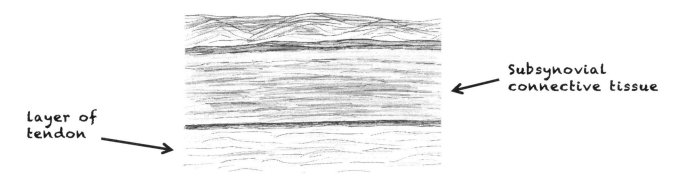

Figure 13. The subsynovial connective tissue which sits on and attaches to the tendons in the carpal tunnel.

And here are the changes that have been found to take place in the subsynovial connective tissue in people with carpal tunnel syndrome…

- samples of subsynovial connective tissue were taken from 11 patients with idiopathic carpal tunnel syndrome and 14 cadavers with no history of carpal tunnel (Ettema 2006). Using an electron microscope, researchers found that the people with carpal tunnel had *much thicker* subsynovial connective tissue than the controls. These findings have also been repeated in other studies (Oh 2006).

Even more interesting is that researchers can reproduce these kinds of changes in experiments…

- 14 rabbits had wires tied around their wrist area to increase carpal tunnel pressure and restrict blood flow (Lluch 1992). After keeping the wires on for various periods of time (from one to three weeks), the subsynovial connective tissue started to thicken. It was noted that the longer the wires were left on, the more thickening occurred. Poor bunny!

So apparently people with carpal tunnel syndrome can have much thicker tissue around the nine tendons that sit in their carpal tunnel – which of course takes up more space in the carpal tunnel – and in turn drives pressure up *even* further. This would help explain why people who have carpal tunnel syndrome have higher carpal tunnel pressures – even when they're *resting* their hands with the wrist out straight (Sanz 2005, Luchetti 1998).

So What Causes Carpal Tunnel Syndrome?

You should now have a better idea of what can cause the symptoms of carpal tunnel syndrome. While the short answer is "increased pressure in the carpal tunnel", there are several effects of this increased pressure that can take place. On the following page is a diagram summarizing the possible pathways that can occur to give someone carpal tunnel syndrome.

people with carpal tunnel syndrome many times
have smaller than normal carpal tunnels

wrist extension and flexion
makes the carpal tunnel smaller

repeated gripping, holding objects, and
pressing the fingers against resistance

carpal tunnel pressure goes up

blood flow decreases
to the carpal tunnel

blood flow decreases
to the median nerve

median nerve
swelling

ischemic reperfusion injury

median nerve
becomes fibrotic

subsynovial connective
tissue gets thicker

carpal tunnel
symptoms

carpal tunnel
symptoms

carpal tunnel pressure goes up

carpal tunnel
symptoms

Is Surgery the Only Answer?

Interestingly enough, when surgeons do a carpal tunnel release and cut the transverse ligament in the wrist, pressure in the carpal tunnel *immediately* drops, circulation to the nerve *instantly* increases, and symptoms most of the time improve. What does this tell us? Reducing the pressure and improving blood flow to the hand and nerve are a key part of permanently relieving symptoms. And in the pages to follow, I'm going to show you ways of doing this *without* having to cut your transverse ligament.

Quick Review

✓ most cases of carpal tunnel syndrome are called "idiopathic" because no obvious cause can be identified – however the research gives us some pretty good clues as to what is going on

✓ for instance, studies show us that people with carpal tunnel syndrome often times have smaller than normal carpal tunnels - which gives a person less "wiggle room" if any changes occur. This helps explain why one person can, say, type all day and have no symptoms, while the person sitting next to them doing the same thing gets carpal tunnel syndrome.

✓ certain wrist and hand motions are known to increase the pressure in the carpal tunnel – which can decrease the blood flow to the carpal tunnel and the median nerve inside it

✓ on again/off again blood flow to the wrist can cause an ischemic-reperfusion injury – which in turn causes median nerve fibrosis and thickens the subsynovial connective tissue

✓ any or all of these events (decreased blood flow to the median nerve, thicker subsynovial connective tissue, or median nerve fibrosis) can cause the symptoms of carpal tunnel syndrome

---

A Quick Tip to Get *Instant* Relief

Yes, it's true, there is a way to get *instant* relief from carpal tunnel symptoms that works in many cases. It goes like this...

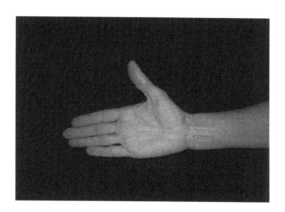

Step #1 – stick your hand with carpal tunnel out - your fingers should be straight

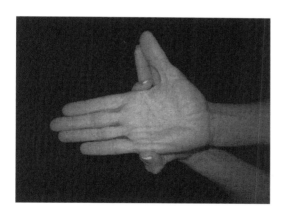

Step #2 – take the thumb and index finger of your *other* hand and put them on the sides of the hand with carpal tunnel – they should be at knuckle level and on the sides of your knuckles

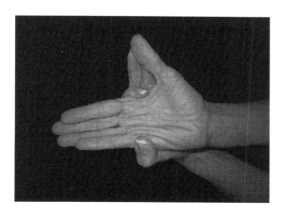

Now gently squeeze. As you do this, symptoms you have in your hand and fingers (such as tingling) should be decreased, or go away entirely.

A few notes. Don't squeeze too hard or this may actually make things worse. Also, make sure the fingers doing the squeezing are on the side of the bony knuckles, like in the picture – putting them too low can make symptoms worse too.

The good news is that, while this technique doesn't work for *every* person with carpal tunnel syndrome, it is successful around 90% of the time. The bad news is that the effects are only temporary – but sometimes symptoms are so bad you'll take what you can get, like when you wake up in the night with pain.

Now if you do find this technique helpful, don't thank me. I found out about it some time ago, buried in a 1999 study in the journal *Muscle and Nerve* (Manente 1999). Why it works nobody is really sure.

Getting Long-Term Relief
Step One: Rest the Nerve

There's no question that the median nerve is taking a beating in carpal tunnel syndrome. It is under more pressure, gets less blood, and can even become fibrotic in some cases. For sure it needs *some rest*.

So just how do you go about resting the median nerve? Well, you put it in a good resting position – one where it's under the lowest pressure and the blood flow is the best. And the research tells us that this ideal position is one where your wrist is *straight* or what a physical therapist would call the *neutral* position. Here's what it looks like...

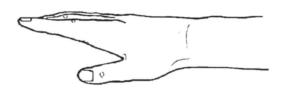

Figure 14. This wrist is in the neutral position.

No, it's not a fancy position, but as far as your median nerve is concerned, it's a vacation! Think about it, in this position, the wrist isn't bent, which we know increases carpal tunnel pressure and slows blood flow – all the things that take its toll on the median nerve.

The problem is, while this is the best position to rest the median nerve, how are we going to keep it in this position for very long?

Splints

Splints are one of the most well-researched tools used to treat carpal tunnel syndrome – and they work….

- this clinical study took took 50 people with carpal tunnel syndrome and randomized them into two groups. Group one wore a splint at night, while the subjects in group two got no treatment (Premoselli 2006). At the end of the 6-month study, subjects who wore the splint had significantly improved compared to the control group.

I also need to point out that this is one of the best kind of studies you can do to prove that a treatment works – subjects were randomized and there was a control group. Furthermore, the control group had *no* treatment, so you can tell if carpal tunnel patients just get better on their own because of Mother Nature.

Yet other research reveals specific effects that splints have on people with carpal tunnel syndrome…

- 10 patients with carpal tunnel syndrome had MRI scans done of their were median nerve and then instructed to wear a splint at night (Schmid 2012). After one week, repeat MRI scans showed that the median nerve was significantly *less swollen*.

You'll notice in both of these studies that subjects wore their splints *only* at night. One wonders though, would wearing it all day be even better? Let's see what the research has to say…

- in this study, subjects were randomized to wear a splint all day and night, or only at night (Walker 2000). Six-weeks later, researchers checked to see which group had the most improvement in symptoms and could use their hands better. Results showed no difference between the two groups.

Looks like whether you wear a splint all day and night, or just at nighttime, well, it seems to makes little difference as far as how your hand feels and moves.

Now that you know all about the benefits of wearing a splint, it's time to figure out which kind to try. When picking one out, make sure it meets these two requirements:

- it keeps your wrist in a neutral position

- it is comfortable enough for you to be able to wear at night (or longer if you choose to)

So you don't need anything fancy. Here's a few pictures of what your typical off the shelf splint looks like. It uses velcro to keep it in place, and can be found at most drugstores.

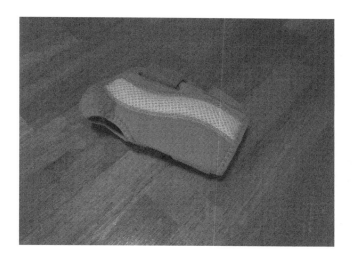

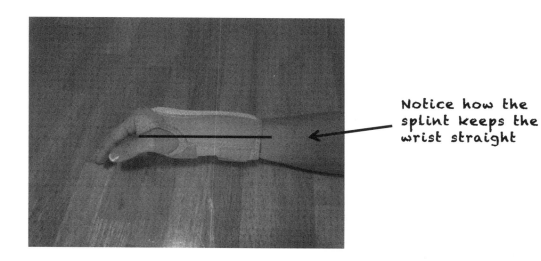

Notice how the splint keeps the wrist straight

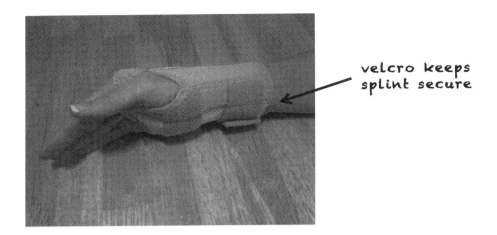

velcro keeps
splint secure

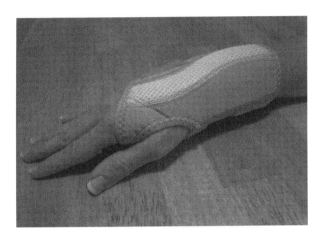

Quick Review

✓ the first step in getting relief from carpal tunnel is to rest the median nerve

✓ the best way to rest it is to put it in a *neutral* position - in this position, the pressure on it is low and blood flow to it is good

✓ wearing a splint at night has been proven to decrease median nerve swelling and get rid of the symptoms of carpal tunnel

✓ choose a splint that is comfortable to wear and keeps your wrist in a neutral position

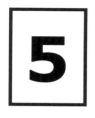

Step Two: Increase the Circulation to the Nerve

Now that we're using the splint to take stress off the median nerve and give it a rest, the next step is to boost its circulation as much as possible. By bringing more blood to the area of the median nerve, an area we know has circulation problems, we are speeding up any healing that needs to take place. Be aware that the time it takes for something to heal *largely* depends on how good the blood supply is to the injured area, for instance...

- it is a known fact that diabetics can take longer to heal because of their poor circulation

- cuts in areas that have a bigger blood supply heal quicker – a cut on your face generally heals faster than a cut on your toe.

- wrist fractures are known to be some of the slowest healing broken bones due to their poor blood supply – compare this to a broken thigh bone that has lots of vascular muscle around it

So how do you go about improving the circulation to your wrist and carpal tunnel area? Well, the first way is pretty simple - by applying *heat* – and its been shown to really help people with carpal tunnel syndrome...

- in this short-term study, people with wrist pain (some of which had carpal tunnel syndrome) were randomized to try a heat wrap, an unheated wrap, a fake pain pill, or a real pain pill (Michlovitz 2004). The heat wrap was worn around the wrist area for 8 hours a day. After three days, the carpal tunnel patients who used the heat wrap had significantly less pain, less stiffness, and increased grip strength compared to carpal tunnel patients who took the fake pain pill.

The carpal tunnel patients in the above study who got such fantastic benefits from using heat (in only three days no less) used a wrap similar to this...

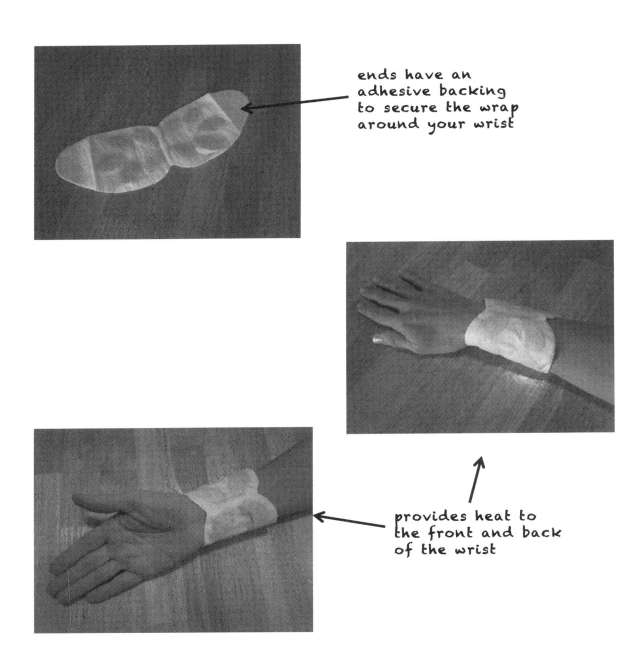

ends have an
adhesive backing
to secure the wrap
around your wrist

provides heat to
the front and back
of the wrist

Heat wraps such as these usually come in a pack of three or so and last from 8 to 12 hours depending on the brand- and can be found in most drug stores. They do a great job in providing continuous heat to the wrist area, which has shown to decrease symptoms a lot.

Alternative ways to apply heat to your wrist? Well, while it's not practical to wear on your wrist all day, you can always try an *electric heating pad*. And if you don't have one of those, there is a cheaper way to go – make your own hot pack. All you'll need are three things:

a cotton tube sock...

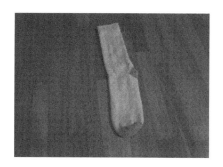

...a bag of regular white rice

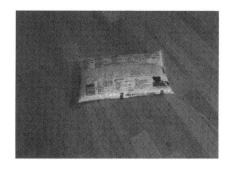

...and a microwave

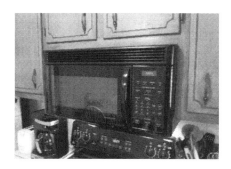

So here's what you do. Fill the cotton sock about ¾ of the way full of the rice. Make sure it's regular, uncooked white rice, and *not* instant or minute rice. This ordinary tube sock has been filled with a whole 2-pound bag of rice, but vary the amount as you see fit...

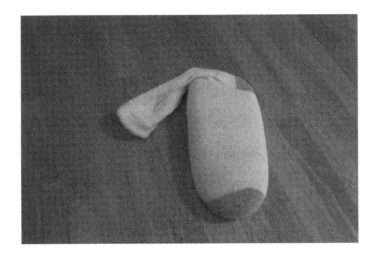

Next, tie off the top – it will look like this when you're finished...

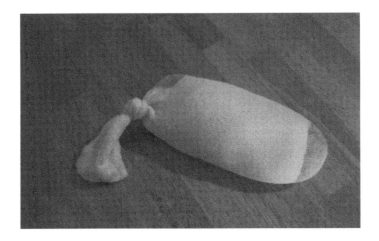

Now all you've got left to do is just pop it into the microwave and heat it up...

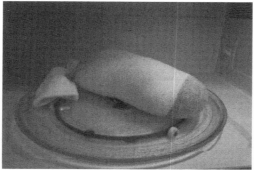

So how long do you stick it in for? Well, that depends how hot you want it. It's going to be a trial and error kind of thing, so I recommend heating it up for one minute the first time, and then carefully checking the temperature to see if that's hot enough for your liking. If not, put it back in for another minute and re-test.

Now when you have the rice sock heated up to your ideal temperature, put the sock wherever the heat feels the best on your wrist, several times a day for 10 to 20 minutes - whether it be on the top of your hand, the bottom of your hand, or sandwiched in between...

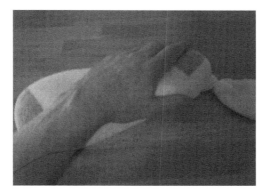

While applying heat to the hand is generally pretty safe for most people, there are certain medical conditions where feeling the heat can be a problem, such as with diabetic individuals – and one could possibly get burned. This is why I recommend everyone check with their doctor before trying out the heat - just to make sure its okay.

The second way you can use to increase the circulation to the wrist area is by *massaging* it. Once again, I'm only going to suggest treatments that the research has shown to actually work...

- 16 adults with carpal tunnel symptoms were randomized to one of two groups (Field 2004). Subjects in group one got a once a week massage and were taught how to massage their own hand and forearm daily. Subjects in group two got no treatment. After four weeks, subjects in the massage group had lower pain levels and increased grip strength compared to the control group.

This study in particular caught my attention because the subjects got better by using just massage – most of which was self-massage! Talk about an economical and effective treatment.

So is it hard to give yourself an effective massage to increase the circulation to your wrist and lessen carpal tunnel symptoms? Not really. In fact one of my favorite massage/carpal tunnel studies (Madenci 2012) got it down to an art – they created an effective 5-step self-massage for carpal tunnel syndrome patients – which takes a whole three minutes to perform! I've detailed the steps on the next page...

Step One

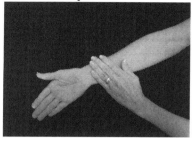

Start out by rubbing your wrist area lightly for 30 seconds using upward strokes (towards the elbow)

Step Two

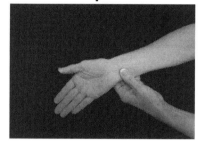

Then use your thumb to make little clockwise circles over the wrist area for 60 seconds.

Step Three

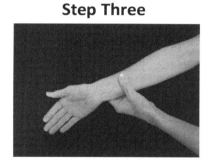

Next, use your thumb to rub the wrist area firmly using upward (towards the elbow) strokes for 30 seconds.

Step Four

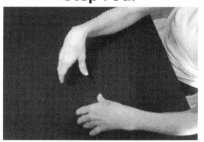

Now shake both of your hands for 30 seconds.

Step Five

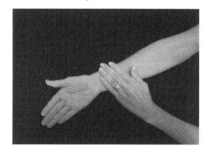

End by rubbing your wrist area lightly for 30 seconds using upward strokes (same as in Step 1).

So what did you think? If for some reason if doesn't appeal to you, or the mechanics of it just don't work out, I do have an alternative massage method you can try – it uses a tennis ball...

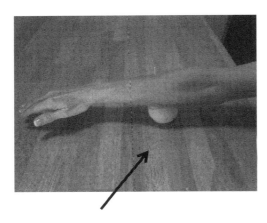

Take a tennis ball and put it under your forearm.

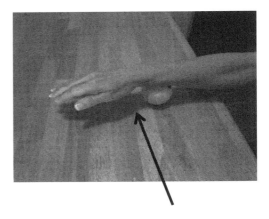

Roll the ball down to your wrist. Then roll it back up to your elbow - repeat this for several minutes.

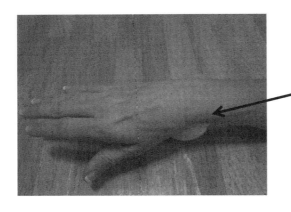

After working the forearm, place the ball under your wrist, and make little circles for a few more minutes.

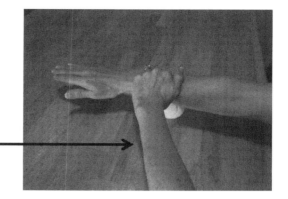

Use your other arm and lean into it a little if you feel like you need a little more pressure, like this...

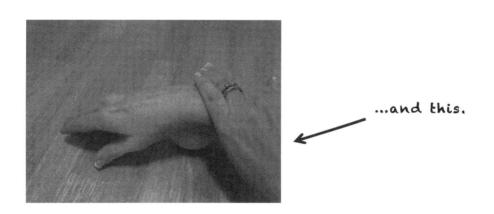

...and this.

And that's it! The vast majority of studies that have shown massage to be effective have had people do it *daily*. Now that you've got a few good tools at your disposal, use them to help increase the circulation to your carpal tunnel and median nerve areas – and you can do them just about anywhere. On to Step Three...

Quick Review

✓ the better the blood flow is to an area of the body, the faster it heals

✓ heat is one good way to improve blood flow to an area and has been shown to decrease the symptoms of carpal tunnel syndrome

✓ massage is also another good way to improve circulation to an area – many studies have shown massage to positively lessen the symptoms of carpal tunnel syndrome

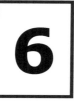

Step Three: Lower Pressure In the Carpal Tunnel

There is no question that people with carpal tunnel syndrome have higher than normal pressure in their carpal tunnel, which creates a lot of problems for the median nerve that lies within it. Therefore, getting the pressure down is essential. Surgeons cut the transverse ligament, the "roof" of the carpal tunnel, to drastically lower the pressure – but is there another way?

Actually there is. Right here, right now, sitting in a chair, I can show you a way that's been *scientifically proven* to lower the pressure in your carpal tunnel – and keep it there for *at least* fifteen minutes. Ready? Okay, just follow the pictures...

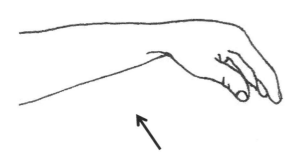

Stick your arm out like this.

Now bend your wrist and fingers straight up...

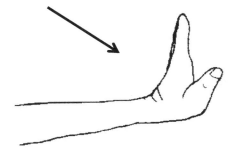

...and then curl your wrist and fingers down making a fist...

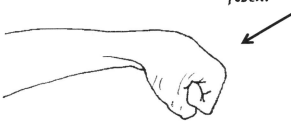

...and bend your wrist and fingers straight up again.

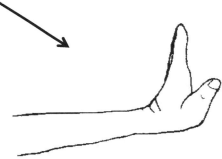

- repeat this up and down wrist motion for 1 minute
- how fast should you go? 2 seconds up, 2 seconds down

At this point, some readers might be a bit confused. In Chapter 2, the book said wrist flexion and extension makes carpal tunnel pressure go *up* – so how can these motions make it go *down*?

The answer is because it's done repeatedly for only a minute. On the other hand, if you kept doing these motions for fifteen minutes, or all day long off and on, they would have a *totally* different effect on the wrist – they would overstress it.

Think if it like weight lifting – if you go to the gym and do one set of the bench press, it can make you stronger - and it's a good thing. Now if you do bench presses *all* day long, it becomes harmful – even though it's *the exact* same exercise that could make you stronger. The key? A little bit of the *right* kind of stress is productive – too much can get you into trouble.

If you're still worried, well, like everything in this book, we have some good research to prove that it actually works in carpal tunnel sufferers...

- this study involved 92 patients with carpal tunnel syndrome and 21 control subjects without it (Seradge 1995). Among other activities, researchers had all subjects active flex and extend their wrists and fingers for one minute. The pressure in the carpal tunnel was measured before and after. Results showed that the carpal tunnel pressure dropped significantly for 15 minutes after the exercise was stopped – *in both patients and controls.*

This was a pretty impressive study. The average resting pressure in the carpal tunnel in patients was 44 mmHg (millimeters of mercury – the same way your blood pressure is measured). After one minute of wrist flexion and extension, pressure dropped to 25 mmHg for fifteen minutes - wow! And for all we know, it might stay down even longer after the one minute of exercise – but this was never tested.

So just how many times a day should you do it? Well, as we've discussed, too much of a good thing can do harm. Since everybody is a little different, you'll have to use a little trial and error at first.

The goal of the exercise is to temporarily drop the pressure in the carpal tunnel – which gives things a chance to "catch-up" and heal as the stress is taken off the median nerve. So, I would start out by doing it three times a day, say morning, noon, and night. If it seems to aggravate your symptoms (not likely), do it less. On the other hand, if things are going well, try working up to doing the 1-minute exercise every couple of hours or so. Isn't it always the simplest things that seem to work the best?

Quick Review

✓ increased carpal tunnel pressure creates a lot of problems for the median nerve – so lowering it is of primary importance

✓ it *is* possible to drop the pressure in the carpal tunnel for at least 15 minutes by doing the 1-Minute wrist exercise – this creates an opportunity for things to "catch-up" and heal as the stress is taken off the median nerve

✓ start out using the 1-Minute exercise three times a day, and adjust the frequency as needed

---

Tracking Recovery

In this book, I've set up a three-step treatment plan – each step designed to short-circuit a *specific* problem in carpal tunnel syndrome. Here's a summary...

Instant Relief

✓ hand squeeze

Long-Term Relief

Step One: Rest the Nerve

✓ wear a splint at night

Step Two: Increase the Circulation to the Nerve

✓ heat wrap
✓ electric heating pad
✓ rice sock
✓ 5-step self-massage
✓ tennis ball self-massage

Step Three: Lower Pressure in the Carpal Tunnel

✓ 1-Minute Wrist Exercise

Okay. So you've learned all about carpal tunnel syndrome, started the three-step plan, and are on the road to recovery. So now what should you expect?

Well, we all know you should expect to get better. But what exactly does *better* mean? As a physical therapist treating patients, it means two distinct things to me:

- your hand starts to *feel* better

and

- your hand starts to *work* better

And so, when a patient returns for a follow-up visit, I will re-assess them, looking for specific changes in their hand **pain**, as well as their hand **function**.

In this book, I'm going to recommend that readers do the same thing periodically. Why? Simply because people in pain can't always see the progress they're making. For instance, sometimes a person's hand pain doesn't seem to be getting any better, but they can now do some motions or tasks that they couldn't do before - a sure sign that things *are* healing. Or, sometimes a person still has significant hand pain, but they're not looking at the fact that it's actually occurring less frequently - yet another good indication that positive changes are taking place.

Whatever the case may be, if a person isn't looking at the big picture, and doesn't think they're getting any better, they're likely to get discouraged and stop doing their treatment altogether - even though they really might have been on the right track.

On the other hand though, what if you periodically check your progress and are keenly aware that your hand *is* making some changes for the better? What if you can *positively* see *objective* results? My guess is that you're going to be giving yourself a healthy dose of motivation to stick with the plan.

Having said that, I'm going to show you exactly what to check for from time-to-time so that you can monitor the changes that are taking place. I call them "outcomes" and there are two of them.

Outcome #1:
Look for Changes in Your Pain

First of all, you should look for changes in your pain. I know this may sound silly, but sometimes it's my job to get a person to see that their pain *is* actually improving. You see, a lot of people come to physical therapy thinking they're going to be pain-free right away. Then, when they're not instantly better and still having pain, they often start to worry and become discouraged. Truth is, I have yet to treat a patient for carpal tunnel syndrome and have them get instantly better. Better yes, but not *instantly* better.

Over the years, I have found that patients usually respond to treatment in a quite predictable pattern. One of three things will almost always occur as a patient begins to turn the corner and get better...

- your hand symptoms will be just as intense as always, however now they are occurring much less frequently

  or

- your hand symptoms are now *less* intense, even though they are still occurring just as frequently

  or

- you start to notice less symptoms *and* they are now occurring less frequently

The point here is to make sure that you keep a sharp eye out for any of these three changes as you progress with the three-step plan. If *any* of them occur, it will be a sure sign that the plan is helping, and you're on the right track. You can then look forward to the pain gradually getting better, usually over the weeks to come.

Outcome #2:
Look for Changes in Hand Function

Looking at how well your hand works is very important because many times hand function improves *before* the pain does. For example, sometimes a patient will do the plan for a while, and although their hand will still hurt a lot, they are able to do many things that they hadn't been able to in a while - a really good indicator that healing is taking place *and* that the pain should be easing up soon.

While measuring your hand function may sound like a pain in the butt, it doesn't have to be. In this book, I'm recommending that readers use a quick and easy assessment tool known as *The Boston Carpal Tunnel Syndrome Questionnaire.*

While it has a pretty long name, it is a really useful tool you can use to keep track of how your hand is feeling and *functioning*. Studies show that it is a valid (Levine 1993), has good test-retest reliability (Greenslade 2004), and is responsive to clinical changes (Gay 2003). And best of all, *it takes only a couple of minutes to complete*. Now that's my kinda test!

So what exactly does taking the *Boston Carpal Tunnel Syndrome Questionnaire* involve? Not much…

- there are two scales, a functional scale (8 questions), and a symptom scale (11 questions)

- read the instructions on each scale and circle the number that applies

- next, add up the numbers you circled and divide by the number of questions for each scale

On the next several pages are the functional and symptom scales that make up the *Boston Carpal Tunnel Syndrome Questionnaire*, let's have a look….

FUNCTIONAL STATUS SCALE

On a typical day during the past two weeks have hand and wrist symptoms caused you to have any difficulty doing the activities listed below? Please circle one number that best describes your ability to do the activity.

Activity	No Difficulty	Mild Difficulty	Moderate Difficulty	Severe Difficulty	Cannot Do at All Due to Hand or Wrist Symptoms
Writing	1	2	3	4	5
Buttoning of clothes	1	2	3	4	5
Holding a book while reading	1	2	3	4	5
Gripping of a telephone handle	1	2	3	4	5
Opening of jars	1	2	3	4	5
Household chores	1	2	3	4	5
Carrying of grocery bags	1	2	3	4	5
Bathing and dressing	1	2	3	4	5

To get your score, simply add up the numbers you circled and divide by 8.

SYMPTOM SEVERITY SCALE

The following questions refer to your symptoms for a typical twenty-four-hour period during the last two weeks (circle one answer to each question).

How severe is the hand or wrist pain that you have at night?
1 I do not have hand or wrist pain at night
2 Mild pain
3 Moderate pain
4 Severe pain
5 Very severe pain

How often did hand or wrist pain wake you up during a typical night in the past two weeks?
1 Never
2 Once
3 Two or three times
4 Four or five times
5 More than five times

Do you typically have pain in your hand or wrist during the daytime?
1 I never have pain during the day
2 I have mild pain during the day
3 I have moderate pain during the day
4 I have severe pain during the day
5 I have very severe pain during the day

How often do you have hand or wrist pain during the daytime?
1 Never
2 Once or twice a day
3 Three to five times a day
4 More than five times a day
5 The pain is constant

How long, on average, does an episode of pain last during the daytime?
1 I never get pain during the day
2 Less than 10 minutes
3 10 to 60 minutes
4 Greater than 60 minutes
5 The pain is constant throughout the day

Do you have numbness (loss of sensation) in your hand?
1 No
2 I have mild numbness
3 I have moderate numbness
4 I have severe numbness
5 I have very severe numbness

Do you have weakness in your hand or wrist?
1 No weakness
2 Mild weakness
3 Moderate weakness
4 Severe weakness
5 Very severe weakness

SYMPTOM SEVERITY SCALE (continued)

Do you have tingling sensations in your hand?
  1 No tingling
  2 Mild tingling
  3 Moderate tingling
  4 Severe tingling
  5 Very severe tingling

How severe is the numbness (loss of sensation) or tingling at night?
  1 I have no numbness or tingling at night
  2 Mild
  3 Moderate
  4 Severe
  5 Very severe

How often did hand numbness or tingling wake you up during a typical night during the past two weeks?
  1 Never
  2 Once
  3 Two or three times
  4 Four or five times
  5 More than five times

Do you have difficulty with the grasping and use of small objects such as keys or pens?
  1 No difficulty
  2 Mild difficulty
  3 Moderate difficulty
  4 Severe difficulty
  5 Very severe difficulty

To get your score, simply add up the numbers you circled and divide by 11.

So how were your scores? Keep in mind that they will range anywhere from a 1 to a 5 for each scale. Higher scores mean you're in bad shape, so your goal is to score as *low* as possible.

If you did score high though, don't worry. Just keep taking the *Boston Carpal Tunnel Syndrome Questionnaire* every few weeks, and as you make progress, you will see your score go lower and lower as time passes. Remember, sometimes hand function gets better *before* the pain does.

Quick Review

✓ being aware of your progress is an important part of treating your carpal tunnel syndrome – it motivates you to keep doing the three-step treatment plan

✓ look for the pain to become less *intense*, less *frequent*, or both to let you know that the three-step plan is working

✓ sometimes your hand starts to work better *before* it starts to feel better. Taking the *Boston Carpal Tunnel Syndrome Questionnaire* from time-to-time makes you aware of improving hand function (and symptoms).

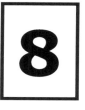

How to *Prevent* Carpal Tunnel Syndrome

When your carpal tunnel syndrome is gone, you certainly won't want it to come back, ever again. And that's the whole purpose of this chapter – to teach you how to *prevent* carpal tunnel syndrome from re-occurring. But is this really possible? Absolutely. Here's a good example from the literature...

- this study sought to try and prevent carpal tunnel syndrome from occurring in a meat packing company with 286 workers (Seradge 2000). In 1997, the company had 55 cases of carpal tunnel syndrome. After making it mandatory that workers perform a short series of exercises before work (taking about 3 minutes), the number of carpal tunnel cases drastically decreased to 22 cases in 1998 – a significant 45% reduction.

So it *is* possible to prevent carpal tunnel syndrome – and it doesn't take a lot of effort either. In the above study, the production workers did a short series of exercise only once a day – before they started working. Essentially, it worked like a "warm-up" for their hands and wrists, preparing them for the repetitive tasks to come – and obviously it made a big difference. On the following pages are some of the exercises that the workers did in the study...

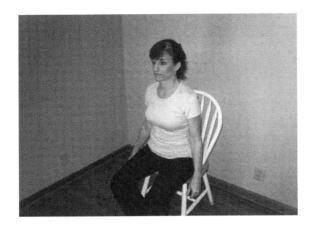

Exercises can be done sitting or standing. Do at the beginning and end of the day – and every few hours as possible.

Start by shaking arms for a count of 10.

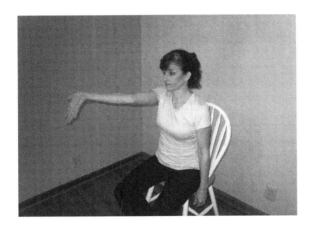

Now lift one of your arms to shoulder level, palm up. Spread fingers and gently bend wrist until fingers point to the floor. Hold for a count of 10.

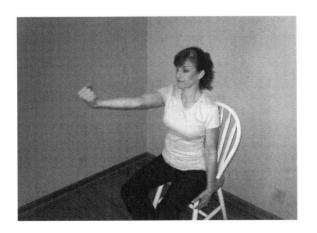

Next, bring fingers and wrist up, forming a tight fist. Bend wrist towards you while keeping elbow straight. Hold for a count of 10.

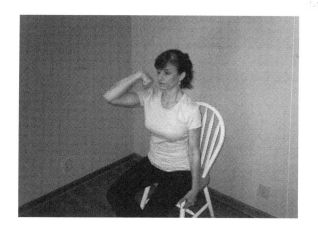

Now bend your elbow pulling your fist to your shoulder. Hold for a count of 10.

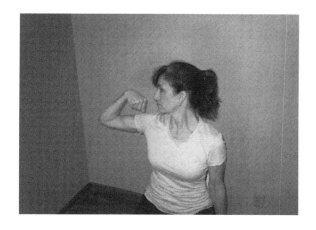

Next, rotate arm out to your side keeping elbow bent and fist held - then slowly turn your head to your fist. Hold for a count of 10.

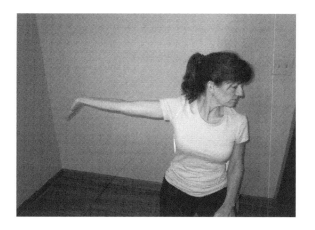

Lastly, you're going to straighten your elbow and fingers and bend your wrist - pointing fingers to floor.

Then slowly turn head to the opposite shoulder. Hold for a count of 10.

Repeat with other arm. Once you're familiar with all the steps, doing both arms should take you just a few minutes to do.

In case that series doesn't appeal to you, a good alternative is the 1-Minute exercise from Chapter 6. It's been proven to lower carpal tunnel pressure - and will thus give your median nerve a nice break throughout the day.

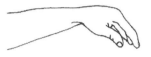 Stick your arm out like this.

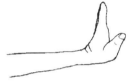 Bend wrist and fingers up.

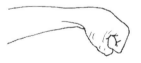 Curl wrist and fingers down.

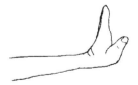 Bend wrist and fingers up again. Repeat this up and down motion for 1 minute at a pace of 2 seconds up and 2 seconds down.

So there you have it, two series of exercises you can do just about anywhere in sitting or standing. Try doing them frequently throughout the day. Like they say, an ounce of prevention is worth a pound of cure!

Quick Review

✓ it is entirely possible to prevent carpal tunnel syndrome

✓ brief wrist and arm exercise has been shown to be an effective tool in preventing carpal tunnel syndrome in the work environment

✓ it is recommended to do the exercises before you start working, and frequently throughout the day, as possible

---

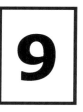 # List of Supporting References

It's true! All the information in this book is based on randomized controlled trials and scientific studies that have been published in peer-reviewed journals. Since I know there are readers out there that like to actually check out the information for themselves, I've included the references for every study I have cited in this book...

Chapter 2

Cudlip S, et al. Magnetic resonance neurography studies of the median nerve before and after carpal tunnel decompression. *J Neurosurg* 2002;96:1046-1051.

Dekel S, et al. Idiopathic carpal tunnel syndrome caused by carpal stenosis. *British Medical Journal* 1980 280;1297-1299.

Ettema A, et al. Changes in the functional structure of the tenosynovium in idiopathic carpal tunnel syndrome: a scanning electron microscope study. *Plast Reconstr Surg* 2006;118:1413-1422.

Freeland A, et al. Biochemical evaluation of serum and flexor tenosynovium in carpal tunnel syndrome. *Microsurgery* 2002;22:378-385.

Gelmers HJ. Primary carpal tunnel stenosis as a cause of entrapment of the median nerve. *Acta Neurochirurgica* 1981;55:316-320.

Guan J, et al. Sonographic and electrophysiological detection in patients with carpal tunnel syndrome. *Neurological Research* 2011;33:970-975.

Horch R, et al. Median nerve compression can be detected by magnetic resonance imaging of the carpal tunnel. *Neurosurgery* 1997;41:76-83.

Lluch A. Thickening of the synovium of the digital flexor tendons: cause or consequence of the carpal tunnel syndrome? *Journal of Hand Surgery* 1992;17B:209-212.

Luchetti R, et al. Correlation of segmental carpal tunnel pressures with changes in hand and wrist positions in patients with carpal tunnel syndrome and controls. *Journal of Hand Surgery* 1998;23B:498-602.

Oh J, et al. Morphological changes of collagen fibrils in the subsynovial connective tissue in carpal tunnel syndrome. *Journal of Bone and Joint Surgery* 2006;88A:824-831.

Ozcan H, et al. Dynamic doppler evaluation of the radial and ulnar arteries in patients with carpal tunnel syndrome. *Am J Roentgenol* 2011;197:W817-20.

Papaioannou T, et al. Carpal canal stenosis in men with idiopathic carpal tunnel syndrome. *Clinical Orthopaedics and Related Research* 1992;285:210-213.

Sanz J, et al. Postoperative changes of carpal canal pressure in carpal tunnel syndrome: a prospective study with follow-up of 1 year. *Journal of Hand Surgery* 2005;30B:611-614.

Seradage H, et al. In vivo measurement of carpal tunnel pressure in the functioning hand. *Journal of Hand Surgery* 1995;20A:855-859.

Sernik R, et al. Ultrasound features of carpal tunnel syndrome: a prospective case-control study. *Skeletal Radiol* 2008;37:49-53.

Tucci M, et al. Biochemical and histological analysis of the flexor tenosynovium in patients with carpal tunnel syndrome. *Biomed Sci Instrum* 1997;33:246-51.

Tuncali D, et al. Carpal tunnel syndrome: comparison of intraoperative structural changes with clinical and electrodiagnostic severity. *British Journal of Plastic Surgery* 2005;58:1136-1142.

Uchiyama S, et al. Quantitative MRI of the wrist and nerve conduction studies in patients with idiopathic carpal tunnel syndrome. *J Neurol Neurosurg Psychiatry* 2005;76:1103-1108.

Yoshioka S, et al. Changes in carpal tunnel shape during wrist motion. MRI evaluation of normal volunteers. *Journal of Hand Surgery* 1993;18B:620-623.

Chapter 3

Manente G, et al. A relief maneuver in carpal tunnel syndrome. *Muscle & Nerve* 1999;22:1587-1589.

Chapter 4

Premoselli S, et al. Neutral wrist splinting in carpal tunnel syndrome: a 3- and 6- month clinical and neurophysiologic follow-up evaluation of night-only splint therapy. *Europa Medicophysica* 2006;42:121-126.

Schmid A, et al. Effect of splinting and exercise on intraneural edema of the medina nerve in carpal tunnel syndrome – an MRI study to reveal therapeutic mechanisms. *J Orthop Res* 2012;30:1343-1350.

Walker W, et al. Neutral wrist splinting in carpal tunnel syndrome: a comparison of night-only versus full-time wear instructions. *Arch Phys Med Rehabil* 2000;81:424-9.

Chapter 5

Field T, et al. Carpal tunnel syndrome symptoms are lessened following massage therapy. *Journal of Bodywork and Movement Therapies* 2004;8:9-14.

Madenci E, et al. Reliability and efficacy of the new massage technique on the treatment in the patients with carpal tunnel syndrome. *Rheumatol Int* 2012;32:3171-3179.

Michlovitz S, et al. Continuous low-level heat wrap therapy is effective for treating wrist pain. *Arch Phys Med Rehabil* 2004;85:1409-16.

Chapter 6

Seradage H, et al. In vivo measurement of carpal tunnel pressure in the functioning hand. *Journal of Hand Surgery* 1995;20A:855-859.

Chapter 7

Gay R, et al. Comparative responsiveness of the disabilities of the arm, shoulder, and hand, the carpal tunnel questionnaire, and the SF-36 to clinical change after carpal tunnel release. *Journal of Hand Surgery* 2003;28A:250-254.

Greenslade J, et al. DASH and Boston questionnaire assessment of carpal tunnel syndrome outcome: what is the responsiveness of an outcome questionnaire? *Journal of Hand Surgery* 2004;29B:159-164.

Levine D, et al. A self-administered questionnaire for the assessment of severity of symptoms and functional status in carpal tunnel syndrome. *Journal of Bone and Joint Surgery* 1993;75-A:1585-1592.

Chapter 7

Seradge H, et al. Preventing carpal tunnel syndrome and cumulative trauma disorder: effect of carpal tunnel decompression exercises: an Oklahoma experience. *J Oklahoma State Med Assoc* 2000;93:150-153.

Printed in Great Britain
by Amazon

16560530R00041